Medicinal Plants: Beginner's Guide to Organic Medicinal Plants and Herbs

Know Grow and Use These Herbs

Steven Clark

I0423520

TOC

- Marijuana
- Oregano
- Cardamom
- Hawthorn

Cancer

- Blood Root
- Cannabis
- Curcumin
- Echinacea

Infections

- Wild Quinine
- Navajo Tea
- Calendula
- Usnea

Common Cold and Flu

- Elderberry
- Horse Radish
- Ginger
- Garlic

Conclusion

INTRODUCTION

Plants have long been the foundation of medical treatments throughout much of our human history. Modern medicine has recognized that herbalism, a form of alternative medicine since its practice is not strictly based on scientific analysis. It nonetheless recognizes is as a very important part of any medical treatment regime. Yes, there are some plants that will have some unpleasant side-effects which can be made worse when coupled with some prescription medications, but are still just as effective.

Modern medicine has even instituted treatments for diseases such as cancers with many plant based treatments. The World Health Organization (WHO) has stated that about 80% of Asian and African countries use plant medicine as their primary health care, with great success.

With all this in mind, here we present you with some plant medicinal remedies for common ailments. We hope you find them to be useful.

Geranium Leaves

Geranium is scientifically called as Pelagronium Odorantissimum. It is more popularly known for its extensive use in aromatherapy. Many essential oil products made from the Geranium plant are now available on the market with numerous health applications. However, one of the least popular benefits of this plant is the magnificent results to be seen when used as a hair product.

It's applications and benefits include:

Regulation of Sebum Secretion

The sebaceous glands located on our scalps regulate the secretion of sebum, which either makes our hair dry when there is too little or oily when there is too much. What geranium does is balance the presence of this oil in our hair and in our scalps, maximizing the vitality of each strand. As a result, we end up having smooth and silky hair that bounces.

- Promotes hair growth while preventing hair loss.

Hair loss plagues both men and women for different reasons. Nevertheless, whether it is genetic or not, geranium can be used to impede the loss while promoting healthy growth. Due to the fact that it balances the secretion of sebum, it also helps to nourish the scalp. A healthy scalp means healthy hair growth with minimized hair loss.

Dandruff Treatment

Dandruff is one of the most unsightly nuisances to plague the hair. While nourishing the scalp, the essential oil to be found in geranium helps to prevent dandruff from presenting itself. The aroma of the plant gives a big plus.

Of course you could go ahead and buy the essential oil products available, but if you would prefer to save a few dollars then go ahead and pick a few geranium leaves. You can even take to growing the plant in your back yard garden so you have a steady supply.

When using geranium leaves you can mix it with 2 tablespoons of vinegar, half a cup of water and blend it into a paste. Apply this paste as you an intensive hair treatment and leave in your hair for up to 15 minutes.

Or, you could boil the leaves then leave them to soak overnight. Then use your regular shampoo to wash your hair and the geranium water to rinse- as a substitute to regular hard water.

 Do this at least once per week and you will see a big difference.

Aloe Vera

The many benefits of the aloe Vera plant (aloe barbadensis) can be traced back to it 75 known nutrients.

- The benefits for hair care include:
- Scalp itching relief.
- Reduction of scalp redness and inflammation.
- Strengthens and adds luster to your hair.
- Balances the pH of your hair.

- Promotes hair growth.
- Alleviates dandruff with its anti- fungal properties.
- Helps your hair to retain water and moisture.

All these benefits are made possible by both the proteolitic enzymes found in the aloe Vera plant and couple with the respective nutrients. With regards to hair conditioning, aloe vera has an abundance of keratin - the same nutrient which is harnessed and an essential in almost all hair products.

To use aloe vera simply cut its leaf stalks into two- along its length- and apply the gel like substance. Take care to ensure it doesn't get into your eyes, if so rinse immediately. It is also very bitter to taste, as a result you might want to avoid the mouth as well.

Banana

Rich, ripe and absolutely delicious- bananas are easily found all year round with a host of health benefits.

Banana is rich in potassium, carbohydrates, natural oils, Vitamins B6 & C. All these helps to produce benefits to the hair including:

- Protection of the natural elasticity of the hair and preventing split ends.
- Produces a manageable shine and promotes growth.
- Controls dandruff
- One of the best hair loss fighters.

To use banana to tap into these benefits, mash it into a smooth paste and apply generously to your hair- massage it into your scalp. Leave it in for up to 15 minutes. There are some who will cite difficulty with rinsing it out of the hair, however, this is only so if your paste has lumps. Ensure it is smooth and almost liquid. Add a tiny bit of water if it helps.

Hibiscus Flower

Hibiscus is sometimes called the 'flower of hair care'. Each part of the plant is used in a different way for different results. There are also several methods to produce oils, conditioners and shampoos from this plant at home. Since it is also a natural ingredient it is safe for all hair types.

The benefits of using the Hibiscus flower for hair treatments include:

- Preventing split ends.
- Eradicating dandruff.
- Alleviating dryness and dullness of your hair.
- Volumizing and preventing graying of the hair.

To produce the oil:

- Grind 7-8 hibiscus flowers and equal number of leaves.
- Heat a 3/4 cup of any natural oil - coconut or olive oil- in a deep pan.
- When the oil is hot add the grinded mixture, turn the fire off and cover the pan.

- Let it stay covered until it is cool then apply to the hair and scalp and rinse after 15 minutes with hibiscus shampoo or a mild shampoo.

To make hair mask:

- Grind a few hibiscus leaves into a fine paste. DO NOT use water unless absolutely necessary.
    - Mix the paste with half a bowl of unsweetened curd.
- Apply to the roots of your hair for an hour, and then rinse with hibiscus shampoo. This helps to strengthen your hair.

To make shampoo:

- Grind 10-12 hibiscus leaves then add a few drops of your preferred natural oil.

Use this instead of your regular shampoo. It will both rinse the scalp and increase hair growth.

To make conditioner:

- Grind 8-10 hibiscus flowers and enough water to make a paste.

- Ensure the hair is not completely wet when you apply it, since it is meant to act as a deep conditioner.
- Leave in your hair for about an hour then rinse with warm water.

Diabetes

If you are living with diabetes or probably have been diagnosed with pre-diabetes then you will be well aware that maintaining a good nutrition is the most important factor in achieving good health. The foods that you choose as well as physical activity will make a big difference in your daily health.

Here are four natural diabetes control aids to include in your diet.

Banana

There has been a lot of doom and gloom surrounding diabetics and bananas due to its high carbohydrate content as well as glycemic index. Nevertheless, researchers have found that banana in moderation does help with people suffering from low blood sugar.

The high healthy carbohydrate-count promotes glucose in the blood and encourages the pancreas to produce more insulin.

For people with low blood sugar levels, bananas are an excellent addition to their diet.

If you have a high blood sugar level the pairing bananas with proteins such as yogurts or eggs can help prevent blood sugar spikes, while delivering the same healthy carbohydrate that your body can use.

Dandelion

Dandelions are common placed and are often referred to as weeds, despite the fact that their leaves and roots are extremely rich in vitamins and edible.

Dandelions, when consumed, help to normalize blood sugar levels as well as improve cholesterol. Both of these in turn improve diabetic symptoms. The Journal of Ethno pharmacology reported in 2001 that a study was performed where diabetic patients were treated with dandelion extract which lowered blood sugar.

To use:

- Leave some dandelion leaves and roots to dry and then steep them in hot water. Drink as tea up to three times per day.

Note however that in some rare cases, the dandelion tea can cause heartburn.

Greek Clover

This is an annual herb also known as Fenugreek and commonly used in curry. It has aromatic seeds which serve a myriad of medical purposes which include lowering the levels of glucose in the body. This in turn helps to control diabetes. It is also known to lower serum cholesterol and triglycerides found in fat cells.

To use:

- Dry your Greek clover seeds then pound them into a powdered form.
- Mix this powder into warm milk or your preferred green tea and drink at least two times each day.

The seeds can also be eaten wholly just as regularly.

Bitter Gourd

The most vital among the plant medicine control of diabetes is probably bitter gourd. It contains an insulin-like/ hypoglycemic compound which is known as 'plant insulin'. This compound has been proven to lower the sugar levels both in blood and urine, making bitter gourd an excellent anti-diabetes agent.

To use:

- Juice bitter gourd fruits in a juicer or extract the juice from blending it with water, and drink a glass each morning.
- If the mix is not palatable for you, then go ahead and mix it with something tastier.

Melon juice goes perfectly with bitter gourd juice.

Ulcers

Stomach and oral ulcers can be extremely painful and persistent. These ulcers, and especially the stomach ulcers, are cause by the bacteria Helicobacter pylori, which causes the release of ammonia and the formation of ulcers.

In extreme cases hospitalization can occur due to ulcers; however here are four natural remedies for the prevention and treatment of ulcers.

Licorice Root

Also known as Glycyrrhiza glabra, licorice root is one of the most extensively investigated herbs, with medicinal applications in both Western and Eastern medicine.

It is very soothing to irritated mucous membranes and has been used to promote the healing of peptic ulcers. Dr. Michael Murray, one of the authors of The Encyclopedia of Natural Medicine, points out that it works differently from other ulcer drugs. He states that licorice root stimulates the body's normal defense mechanisms to prevent ulcer formation, by increasing the number of mucus-producing cells. By improving the mucus producing cells, the quality of mucus is increased; this then increases the life span of intestinal cells and thus the blood supply to the lining of the intestine. All this helps to cure ulcers as well as prevent their formation.

To use:

- Boil licorice root and drink as tea at least twice each day.

If you would prefer it in a juice then go ahead and use a juice extractor. It is however advised that you mix it with another fruit juice to make it more enjoyable.

Chamomile

It is no secret that the chamomile plant serves many health purposes of soothing effects. The same is true for ulcers of any kind.

It has a soothing effect on irritated and inflamed mucous membranes. This then increases mucous production which cures ulcers and prevents others from forming.

To use:

The chamomile plant is very popular and can be found almost anywhere.

- Get a few leaves and boil them so that the brew is very strong. Drink a cup in the morning and another at nights before bed.

Most doctors recommend that you drink it two-three times each day.

Chamomile is available in capsules as well as green tea bags. However, if you can get it in its natural form the results will be far better.

Ginger

The antibacterial properties, of ginger make it an excellent ulcer fighting agent. It helps to eliminate the bacteria which cause the formation of ulcers, Helicobacter pylori. It also reduces the excess gastric acid in the stomach, which provides the ulcer cells with the perfect environment to thrive.

To use:

Make a cup of ginger tea at least three times per day. As much as is possible, try to use honey to sweeten and not sugar.

Cabbage

When it comes to ulcer treatments there is one lactic acid food that stands out and is more effect than the rest- cabbage. Cabbage juice has been successfully used to prevent and heal stomach ulcers for decades. It has over a 92% success rate

Doctors also report that patients, who drink a quart of pure cabbage juice each day, cure their ulcers in as little time as five days.

To use:

Blend cabbage with a bit of water and then extract the juice. If you have a juice extractor this is far more effective.

Drink the juice up to three times per day, or as often as possible.

High Blood Pressure

Blood pressure is the measure of force with which blood presses against the walls of the blood vessels, high blood pressure also known as hypertension, results in all kinds of other cardiovascular ailments. this is because it forces the heart to work harder to pump blood throughout the body.

Next to obesity and diabetes it is one of the most common ailments plaguing societies today. If you suffer from on this condition, here are four plant medicine solutions you can try.

Marijuana

The famous and controversial cannabis sativa, which has been taking the world by storm, it has the active ingredient known as THC which makes you feel high and relaxed. It also lowers your blood pressure as one feels more relaxed as well as the blood vessels dilate making the flow of blood easier with less pressure needed. These effects are usually short term, lasting about 3-5 hours at most.

When medical marijuana is prescribed for blood pressure control, it is recommended that it be used every 4-5 hours during your waking hours.

To use:

Most people smoke the plant's dried flowers, stems, seeds and leaves. It can also be included in brownies, cookies and lollipops though the body needs more time to break down THC once it is consumed. Others brew as tea or inhale the vapor.

No matter how you choose to use cannabis, it affects every single organ in your body and has the same effect.

Oregano

Oregano is one of those herbs popularly used in Italian dishes such as pasta, salads and pizzas. It can be eaten fresh or dried, just a matter of preference.

Oregano is a sodium free food and so does not contribute to increasing blood pressure. A diet high in sodium is what generally leads to high blood pressure. Many doctors recommend including oregano in ones diet as it helps to lower and maintain a healthy blood pressure.

To use:

- Pick the leaves from an oregano plant and dry them then crush and add to dishes you cook.

You can also choose to use them green.

Though not a common method of consuming it, you can also boom the oregano, sweeten with honey and drink at least twice per day.

Cardamom

Cardamom owes its origins to India and is often used as a seasoning in South Asian dishes.

It has been proven to have several antioxidant properties and 2001 studies show that powdered cardamom significantly reduces blood pressure.

To use:

The powdered cardamom is readily available in health stores and supermarkets.

- It can be added to just about any dish for more flavor.
- The seeds can also be used in soups and stews.
- When baking you can also include the seeds for more flavor

Hawthorn

This is a traditional Chinese medicine remedy for high blood pressure.

The Hawthorn plant has a whole of benefits to cardiovascular health, including the prevent of blood clot formation, promoting good blood circulation which then reduces ones blood pressure.

To use:

You simply make a tea and sweeten with honey as opposed to sugar.

The pill is also sold in most pharmacies, however as always, the natural form is preferred.

Cancers

Cancer is also known as malignant neoplasm. It refers to a group of diseases characterized by the abnormal growth of body cells, which have the potential to spread and invade other parts of the body.

It used to be that cancer was a death sentence but with advances in both traditional medicine and the growing acceptance of alternative medicinal techniques, the odds have shifted somewhat. Here are four natural remedies that can be coupled with treatment.

Blood Root

Also known as Sanguinaria Canadensis, blood root is a flowering plant native to North America. During spring it has beautiful and delicate white flowers. However, it is the root of the plant that holds the magic in the form of an herbal chemical called Sanguinarine.

There are several studies which detail the effects of Sanguinarine on cancer cells. Nevertheless, the bottom line is that it causes cancer cells to die, while doing absolutely no harm to normal healthy cells.

It does cause nausea on occasions though.

To use:

Boil the root of the plant and drink as tea no less than three times each day.

Cannabis

Here comes the good ole marijuana to the rescue once again.

Cannabis sativa originated in Central Asia and has since spread to other parts of the world. The plant produces cannabinoids which contain resin.

These cannabinoids have a drug like effect on both the nervous system and the immune system. Added to the popular THC, the second most active cannabinoid is CBD, known as cannabidiol which causes the relief of pain and also lowers inflammation without actually causing a high.

CBD is used to treat the side effects of cancer and results in other effects such as:

- blocking cell growth
- preventing the growth of the blood vessels which supply tumors.
- helps to relieve muscle spasms.

To use:

- Many people smoke the dried seeds, flowers, stem and leaves of the cannabis plant.

- It can also be consumed by mixing it with brownies and other pastries.
- Others boil it as tea or inhale its vapor.

Curcumin

Curcumis is the active ingredient in Tumeric and acts as an anti-oxidant which protects the body cells from damage caused by free radicals.

Several research studies also show that curcumin impedes the important molecular pathway necessary for cancer development, growth and spread. It inhibits the formation of cancer causing enzymes.

In short, curcumin is an effective anti-inflammatory agent which can be used alongside cancer treatments and possibly to prevent it.

To use:

- Add the powder to lemonade and other juices you consume throughout the day.

The leaf of the plant can also be boiled and had as tea.

The powder should also be used to season dishes you will cook.

Echinacea

Studies have portrayed this herb as an immuno-enhancing herb since its commercial availability several years ago.

Daily consumption of Echinacea has been proven to help to lower leukemia cells over a period of time.

To use:

Drink the herb as tea at least three times per day.

Infections

An infection of any kind is caused by an invasion of the body by disease-causing organisms, the way they multiple and the reaction of the tissues of the body to the toxins they cause.

Here are four plants that can be used to stem and inhibit the chemical pathways of various infections to which the human body is prone.

Wild Quinine

Wild Quinine owes its origins to the Indian tribes of the Southeastern United States, who used it for medicinal and veterinarian purposes-

It grows to a height of about three feet and small white daisy like flowers which grow in clusters. It has been traditionally used to treat fatigue and any type of gastrointestinal infections. The top most parts of the plant have a ´quinine-like´ bitterness which is used to treat fevers associated with infections- thus the colloquial name, feverfew.

To use:

- Boil herb as tea and drink at least three times per day.

Navajo Tea

Also known as Greenthread and Coyote Plant, this is a daisy like plant which grows in the dry regions of the United States and Hawaii.

It has been used as an anti-inflammatory agent for several years and is particularly good at working as a diuretic and to cure urinary tract infections. Research also shows that it is particularly effective at preventing blood platelets from sticking together thus preventing strokes and heart attacks. It is also a powerful detoxing agent, which makes it particularly effective against infections.

To use:

- Boil as tea and drink at least three times per day.
- Some people also advice mixing it with turmeric to pack a more powerful punch.

Calendula

Also known as Calendula officinalis, this plant is extremely effective at treating infections associated with wounds.

This flower is a powerful anti-inflammatory and microbial agent which is mostly used topically. It is advised that you do not consume this plant. It is not poisonous naturally; however it can make you extremely nauseous.

To use:

- Soak some of the leaves as well as the flowers in hot water, drain the excess water then grind into a paste. Apply topically as needed.
- It is also extremely effective against rashes.

Usnea

When you think of plant medicines that are used for infections, the list would not be complete without the mention of Usnea, also known as Usneabarbata.

This bitter tasting plant is used to treat infections associated with abscesses, coughs, colds, cystitis, sore throat, influenza and any respiratory infections. It also has applications in treating mild cervical dysplasia.

Its absorbent qualities have resulted in it being used in baby diapers and sanitary napkins.

To use:

- Dry the lichen of the plant and steam it as tea two-three times daily.
- Remember to sweeten with honey and not sugar as much as is possible.

Capsules are also available in 100 mg to be taken three times daily; however, as much as possible try to consume it in its natural form.

The Common Cold and Flu

Several human studies have demonstrated that the elderberry plant has significant anti-flu properties. This is largely due to the group of antioxidant flavonoids it contains which binds to the influenza virus and prevents infections.

There is also a study which proves that it had significant effects against the scary H1N1 virus. It showed that elderberry inhibited the proliferation of the virus itself.

To use:

- Simply boil the leaves and flower of the plant, strain, sweeten where necessary and drink as tea.

Horse Radish

Herbalists have long since recommended horseradish for common colds, influenza and lung congestion. It causes an excess production of mucus. This might often be view as the cold or flu worsening, however, this is not the case. The free-flowing mucus signals that your body is ridding itself of bacteria and wastes that result from the flu infection. Do not fuss about it for a few days.

Horseradish is also extremely effective against sinus infections (sometimes also resulting from cold or influenza). Stagnant mucus is generally how sinus infection gets started; it is a breeding ground for bacteria to multiply. A bit of horseradish therapy clears that up almost instantly.

To use:

Have you ever bit into maybe a piece of roast beef and instantly felt like your nose was on fire?

That is the horseradish at work. Horseradish goes to work immediately on the nasal cavity.

All you then need to do is to eat some horseradish once or twice per day.

Ginger

Ginger is known to contain about twelve antiviral substances. It is very effective at treating most symptoms associated with the common cold, including:

- Sore throat
- Inflammation and irritation of the mucus membranes
- Coughing
- Pain, as it has a calming effect

The pathway that ginger takes is that impedes the production of the substances that will cause the full blown effect on cold or influenza. It also contains compounds known as gingerols, theses are natural cough suppressants.

To use:

Drink a strong cup of ginger tea at least three times each day.

Even better is the minute you feel the onset of cold or flu symptoms, start dosing up on ginger.

Garlic

Garlic has long since been hailed for its magnificent healing powers, particularly against infectious diseases like cold or flu. This is due to its immune boosting effects. Fresh garlic in particular is a more that potent antibacterial, anti-fungal and antiviral agent.

Much of garlic´s therapeutic effect comes from its intrinsic sulphur containing compounds, such as alicin- also responsible for its characteristic smell. Other compounds which promote health also include oligosaccharides, selenium, flavonoids and arginine rich proteins.

To use:

If you are feeling a bit brave, you can try holding a crushed clove of garlic in your mouth and breathe in the fumes. If it gets too strong then chew it and swallow with water.

You can also steam garlic with a bit of broccoli and eat.

Or there is the option of boiling the garlic into a kind of tea, sweeten with a bit of honey and drink it. Swallow the pieces of the cloves that are still there.

CONCLUSION

The natural remedies presented in this book are not to be used to replace traditionally prescribed medications, but more to be used alongside them. In the case that you are pregnant or have just done surgery of some sort, please consult your physician before adding these herbs to your medication regime.

Natural plant medicine has long since been used before traditional medicine was developed. Our ancestors for sure had to battle many of the same diseases and infections that now plague us. The fact that the human species has not yet been extinct is a sign as to just how effective these plant medicine therapies have been. We see no reason why they cannot be included in today´s treatments.

If you have truly found value in my publications please take a minute and rate my book, I'd be eternally grateful if you left a review on Amazon. As an independent author I rely on reviews for my livelihood and it gives me great pleasure to see my work is appreciated.

www.ingramcontent.com/pod-product-compliance
Lightning Source LLC
Chambersburg PA
CBHW060443290526
45793CB00002B/547